Technical Brief
Number 16

Decision Aids for Advance Care Planning

Prepared for:
Agency for Healthcare Research and Quality
U.S. Department of Health and Human Services
540 Gaither Road
Rockville, MD 20850
www.ahrq.gov

Contract No. 290-2012-00016-I

Prepared by:
Minnesota Evidence-based Practice Center
Minneapolis, MN

Investigators:
Mary Butler, Ph.D., M.B.A.
Ed Ratner, M.D.
Ellen McCreedy, M.P.H.
Nathan Shippee, Ph.D.
Robert L. Kane, M.D.

AHRQ Publication No. 14-EHC039-EF
July 2014

This report is based on research conducted by the Minnesota Evidence-based Practice Center (EPC) under contract to the Agency for Healthcare Research and Quality (AHRQ), Rockville, MD (Contract No. 290-2012-00016-I). The findings and conclusions in this document are those of the authors, who are responsible for its contents; the findings and conclusions do not necessarily represent the views of AHRQ. Therefore, no statement in this report should be construed as an official position of AHRQ or of the U.S. Department of Health and Human Services.

The information in this report is intended to help health care decisionmakers—patients and clinicians, health system leaders, and policymakers, among others—make well informed decisions and thereby improve the quality of health care services. This report is not intended to be a substitute for the application of clinical judgment. Anyone who makes decisions concerning the provision of clinical care should consider this report in the same way as any medical reference and in conjunction with all other pertinent information, i.e., in the context of available resources and circumstances presented by individual patients.

This report may be used, in whole or in part, as the basis for development of clinical practice guidelines and other quality enhancement tools, or as a basis for reimbursement and coverage policies. AHRQ or U.S. Department of Health and Human Services endorsement of such derivative products may not be stated or implied.

This report may periodically be assessed for the urgency to update. If an assessment is done, the resulting surveillance report describing the methodology and findings will be found on the Effective Health Care Program Web site at: www.effectivehealthcare.ahrq.gov. Search on the title of the report.

This document is in the public domain and may be used and reprinted without permission except those copyrighted materials that are clearly noted in the document. Further reproduction of those copyrighted materials is prohibited without the specific permission of copyright holders.

Persons using assistive technology may not be able to fully access information in this report. For assistance contact EffectiveHealthCare@ahrq.hhs.gov.

> None of the investigators have any affiliation or financial involvement that conflicts with the material presented in this report.

Suggested citation: Butler M, Ratner E, McCreedy E, Shippee N, Kane RL. Decision Aids for Advance Care Planning. Technical Brief No. 16. (Prepared by the Minnesota Evidence-based Practice Center under Contract No. 290-2012-00016-I.) AHRQ Publication No. 14-EHC039-EF. Rockville, MD: Agency for Healthcare Research and Quality. July 2014. www.effectivehealthcare.ahrq.gov/reports/final.cfm.

Preface

The Agency for Healthcare Research and Quality (AHRQ), through its Evidence-based Practice Centers (EPCs), sponsors the development of evidence reports and technology assessments to assist public- and private-sector organizations in their efforts to improve the quality of health care in the United States. The reports and assessments provide organizations with comprehensive, science-based information on common, costly medical conditions and new health care technologies and strategies. The EPCs systematically review the relevant scientific literature on topics assigned to them by AHRQ and conduct additional analyses when appropriate prior to developing their reports and assessments.

This EPC evidence report is a Technical Brief. A Technical Brief is a rapid report, typically on an emerging medical technology, strategy or intervention. It provides an overview of key issues related to the intervention—for example, current indications, relevant patient populations and subgroups of interest, outcomes measured, and contextual factors that may affect decisions regarding the intervention. Although Technical Briefs generally focus on interventions for which there are limited published data and too few completed protocol-driven studies to support definitive conclusions, the decision to request a Technical Brief is not solely based on the availability of clinical studies. The goals of the Technical Brief are to provide an early objective description of the state of the science, a potential framework for assessing the applications and implications of the intervention, a summary of ongoing research, and information on future research needs. In particular, through the Technical Brief, AHRQ hopes to gain insight on the appropriate conceptual framework and critical issues that will inform future research.

AHRQ expects that the EPC evidence reports and technology assessments will inform individual health plans, providers, and purchasers as well as the health care system as a whole by providing important information to help improve health care quality.

We welcome comments on this Technical Brief. They may be sent by mail to the Task Order Officer named below at: Agency for Healthcare Research and Quality, 540 Gaither Road, Rockville, MD 20850, or by email to epc@ahrq.hhs.gov.

Richard Kronick, Ph.D.
Director
Agency for Healthcare Research and Quality

Yen-pin Chiang, Ph.D.
Acting Director
Center for Outcomes and Evidence
Agency for Healthcare Research and Quality

Stephanie Chang, M.D., M.P.H.
Director, EPC Program
Center for Outcomes and Evidence
Agency for Healthcare Research and Quality

William Lawrence, M.D., M.S.
Task Order Officer
Center for Outcomes and Evidence
Agency for Healthcare Research and Quality

Acknowledgments

We thank William Lawrence and Tim Carey, whose comments only improved the report. Thanks also to Jeannine Ouellette and Marilyn Eells for the exceptional editing support.

Key Informants

In designing the study questions, the EPC consulted a panel of Key Informants who represent subject experts and end-users of research. Key Informant input can inform key issues related to the topic of the technical brief. Key Informants are not involved in the analysis of the evidence or the writing of the report. Therefore, in the end, study questions, design, methodological approaches, and/or conclusions do not necessarily represent the views of individual Key Informants.

Key Informants must disclose any financial conflicts of interest greater than $10,000 and any other relevant business or professional conflicts of interest. Because of their role as end-users, individuals with potential conflicts may be retained. The TOO and the EPC work to balance, manage, or mitigate any conflicts of interest.

The list of Key Informants who participated in developing this report follows:

Jon Broyles
Coalition to Transform Advanced Care (C-TAC)
Washington, DC

David English, J.D.
American Bar Association Commission on Law and Aging
University of Missouri School of Law
Columbia, MO

Floyd J. Fowler Jr., Ph.D.
Informed Medical Decisions Foundation
Boston, MA

Joanne Lynn, M.D., M.A., M.S.
Center for Elder Care and Advanced Illness
Altarum Institute
Washington, DC

Robert Pearlman, M.D., M.P.H.
Washington VA National Center for Ethics in Health Care
Seattle, WA

Thaddeus Pope, Ph.D.
Hamline University School of Law
St. Paul, MN

Peg Sandeen, Ph.D., M.S.W.
Death with Dignity
Portland, OR

Peer Reviewers

Prior to publication of the final evidence report, EPCs sought input from independent Peer Reviewers without financial conflicts of interest. However, the conclusions and synthesis of the scientific literature presented in this report does not necessarily represent the views of individual reviewers.

Peer Reviewers must disclose any financial conflicts of interest greater than $10,000 and any other relevant business or professional conflicts of interest. Because of their unique clinical or content expertise, individuals with potential non-financial conflicts may be retained. The TOO and the EPC work to balance, manage, or mitigate any potential non-financial conflicts of interest identified.

The list of Peer Reviewers follows:

Jean Kutner, M.D., M.S.P.H.
Professor, University of Colorado School of Medicine
President, American Academy of Hospice and Palliative Medicine
Denver, CO

Jean Kutner, M.D., M.S.P.H.
Professor, University of Colorado School of Medicine
President, American Academy of Hospice and Palliative Medicine
Denver, CO

Benjamin Levi, M.D., Ph.D., FAAP
Advanced care planning decision aids researcher
Penn State College of Medicine
Hershey, PA

Daniel Matlock, M.D., M.P.H.
Advanced care planning decision aids researcher
Assistant Professor of Medicine, Division of General Internal Medicine
University of Colorado School of Medicine
Aurora, CO

Charles Sabatino, J.D.
Borchard Foundation Center on Law & Aging
Washington, DC

Decision Aids for Advance Care Planning

Structured Abstract

Background. Advance care planning (ACP) honors patients' goals and preferences for future care by creating a plan for when illness or injury prevents adequate communication. ACP can also help patients assess their care options. Less than 50 percent of severely or terminally ill patients have an advance directive in their medical record, and physicians are only about 65 percent accurate in predicting patient preferences. Decision aids can provide a structured approach to informing patients about options and prompting them to document and communicate their preferences.

Purpose. We developed a technical brief on the state of practice and current research for decision aids for adult ACP and to provide a framework for future research and effort.

Methods. We interviewed Key Informants representing clinicians, attorneys, consumer advocates, experts in medical law and ethics, and decision aid researchers and developers. We searched online sources for information about available decision aids and conducted a literature search to identify available research on decision aids for adult ACP as an intervention.

Findings. Numerous decision aids are widely available but not represented in the empirical literature. Of the 16 published studies testing decision aids as interventions for adult ACP, most were proprietary or not openly available to the public. Decision aids tend to be constructed for the general population or for disease-specific conditions for narrower decision choices. Designing decision aids that are responsive to diverse philosophical perspectives and flexible to change as people gain experience with their personal illness courses remains an important concern. Future directions for effort include further research, training of ACP facilitators, dissemination and access, and the potential opportunities that lie in social media or other technologies.

Contents

Background 1
Guiding Questions 4
Methods 5
   Discussion With Key Informants 5
   Gray Literature Search 5
   Published Literature Search 6
   Data Organization and Presentation 7
Findings 8
   Description of Existing Decisions for ACP 8
      Existing Decision Aid Tools (Guiding Question 1) 8
      Context in Which ACP Decision Aids Are Used (Guiding Question 2) 16
   Evidence Map 17
      Current Evidence of ACP Decision Aids (Guiding Question 3) 17
      Evaluating ACP Decision Aids 26
Summary and Implications 29
   Important Issues Raised by the Technology (Guiding Question 4) 29
Next Steps 32
References 34

Tables
Table 1.   Characteristics associated with ACP at various stages 2
Table 2.   Inclusion/exclusion criteria by PICOTS 6
Table 3a. Examples of general ACP tools publicly available on the World Wide Web 10
Table 3b. Examples of ACP tools for those with serious or advanced illness publicly available on the World Wide Web 13
Table 4.   ACP decision aid studies 22
Table 5.   Outcomes examined by ACP decision aid studies 24
Table 6.   Evaluating ACP decision aids 28
Table 7.   Potential outcome measure by stage 33

Figures
Figure 1. Map of health states during which ACP may be considered 2
Figure 2. Article flow diagram 17

Appendixes
Appendix A. Interview Guides for Key Informants
Appendix B. Published Literature Search Strategy
Appendix C. Organization Web sites Searched for Gray Literature
Appendix D. Evidence Tables
Appendix E. Examples of Advance Care Planning Tools That Did Not Meet Definition of Decision Aid

Background

Advance care planning (ACP) can be thought about as a way to inform care choices when the patient cannot express a preference, but it is also a planning tool. Seriously ill patients' preferences regarding life-sustaining interventions depend on their goals for care. Some patients prioritize living longer to achieve life goals, while others may not wish to be kept alive when meaningful recovery or a particular quality of life is no longer possible.[1-3] Religious and spiritual values and beliefs may also affect goals of care.[4,5] Advance planning for future care helps to honor patient preferences and goals should incapacitating illness or injury prevent adequate communication.[6]

This Technical Brief considers decision aids that support the ACP process of decisionmaking for future health care needs. ACP generally has three components: (1) learning about anticipated condition(s) and the options for care, (2) considering those options, and (3) communicating preferences for future care, either orally or in writing. Ideally ACP should be included in general care planning, especially for those with complex needs. ACP can be facilitated by a health care provider but may also rely on self-administered tools or attorney-client discussions[7] that focus on clarifying values and choosing a surrogate decisionmaker to serve when the person is incapacitated.

Decision aids help patients consider options in health care. We define ACP decision aids broadly as a form or a tool that includes a behavioral prompt. Aids should include at least three of the International Patient Decision Aid Standards (IPDAS) criteria: an educational component, a structured approach to thinking about choices, and a means of communicating those choices.[8,9]

An individual's health state at the time of planning determines the type of ACP decisions considered. Figure 1 illustrates a health state map based on quadrants in which we locate several common health states that trigger ACP activities. ACP decisions vary depending on the patient's location on the map, remaining life expectancy, and predictability of end-of-life care needs. Understanding what information to provide to support specific ACP treatment decisions generally improves as a person moves from left to right along this map and familiarity with health states increases. However, some disease states have more predictable trajectories than others, and uncertainty about which health states a person will face may persist.

Figure 1. Map of health states during which ACP may be considered

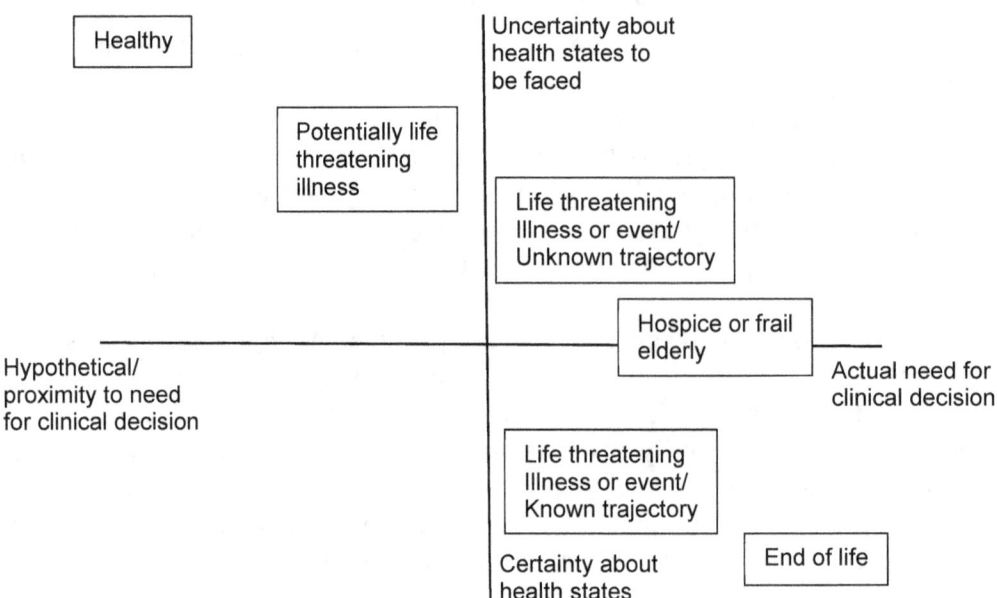

Table 1 outlines how elements of decisionmaking can vary across the Figure 1 map. For example, healthy people may simply identify a proxy decisionmaker and offer some general values and preferences or care goals for various potential events. Those facing potentially life-threatening illness would focus concretely on how to manage emergency care. Those facing serious illness need to think about the likelihood of real benefits from different types of care and interventions and the probability of adverse events from treatment. Correspondingly, the type of information the decisionmaker needs most, and what the decision aid could provide, will vary. Most people gain clarity about what information can best support specific ACP treatment decisions as they move from hypothetical to actual clinical decisions and their familiarity with health states increases, or when the health state for which a decision is needed becomes more certain.

Table 1. Characteristics associated with ACP at various stages

	Stage of Health/Illness			
	Healthy	Potentially Life Threatening Illness	Life Threatening Illness or Event	Hospice or Frail Elderly
Most relevant type of decision within ACP	Naming of proxy decisionmaker	Preferences for emergency management of acute life threatening event	Preferences for ongoing management of chronic illness in event of loss of decisional capacity, use of life support technology	Plan for site of death, preference for sedation versus physical comfort
Setting most common for ACP	Community event, on-line, or with attorney	Health care setting	Health care setting	Health care, hospice
Likelihood of ACP document actually informing an end of life decision	Low	Moderate	High	High
Type of information most needed in ACP decision aid	Role definition for proxy, criteria to consider proxy appropriateness	Probability of adverse event, outcomes with and without life sustaining efforts	Quantity and quality of life for those with advanced chronic illness, disease and intervention-specific benefits vs. burden of life support	Resources available to manage caregiver burden in various settings for end of life care, options for management of acute symptoms

For those not in end-of-life (EOL) situations, ACP decision aids prompt decisions for hypothetical health states they have not yet experienced. This requires people to imagine living with various conditions of disability. Often, however, people have only a tenuous understanding about the health states for which decisions are being made. For example, those imagining hypothetical disabilities consistently view them as more severe than those actually experiencing the disabilities, thus perhaps unknowingly exaggerating their own aversion to living with disability.[10-13] As a result, if treatment-specific decision aids are used early in the Figure 1 map, healthy people may eschew treatment options that, in reality, they might willingly endure. ACP decisions differ from EOL decisions in which the patient tangibly (not hypothetically) experiences the consequences of their choices about treatments.

ACP, particularly among healthy older adults, is often undertaken outside of clinical settings. Nonclinical partners in shared decisionmaking may include other family members, caregivers, or attorneys or other professionals, rather than clinicians. Just as diverse populations are involved in ACP, many formats and types of decision aids are available to help patients and families with ACP. However, the empirical literature supporting decision aids for ACP is sparse, and a recent update of a Cochrane review on decision aids specifically excluded the hypothetical context of ACP decisions.[14]

This Technical Brief presents the "lay of the land" by describing the literature on ACP decision aids and offering a framework to help readers consider which decision aid best meets their needs. Thus, the Brief focuses on the decision aids themselves and the context within which they are used. It does not focus on the ACP decisionmaking process for patients or the tools or forms developed with the sole purpose of documenting advance directives or physician orders. Our Brief is focused solely on adults who are mentally and legally competent, because ACP (and the decision aids that support it) is so complex and encompasses diverse populations with widely varying health states. We excluded discussion of ACP for those who have never had the ability to participate in it, such as individuals with significant developmental disabilities and children. Decisionmaking by parents of gravely ill children differs qualitatively from decisionmaking for adult patients. Further, not only must children as legal minors rely on their parents to make decisions for them, but they may also not reach the age of majority and thus the ability to form their own legally binding decisions.

Opportunity for expansion and improvement of ACP remains. A 2003 Agency for Healthcare Research and Quality literature summary[15] noted that less than 50 percent of the severely or terminally ill patients studied had in their medical records an advance directive, a common outcome of the advance care planning process.[16-19] Further, only 12 percent of patients with an advance directive had received input from their physician in its development,[17] and physicians were only about 65 percent accurate in predicting patient preferences and tended to think patients would want less life-prolonging treatment than they actually desired, even after reviewing the patient's advance directive.[20] Decision aids may improve participation in ACP and the effectiveness of ACP communication by facilitating clear documentation across platforms and providers and by providing insights into why the patients made the decisions they did.

Guiding Questions

The questions we formulated to guide the Technical Brief process are listed below.

1. **What decision aids for ACP have been proposed or used in practice?**
   a. What are the characteristics of the decision aid, such as the goal, mode of delivery, and settings in which it is used?
   b. How well do the decision aids meet decision aid criteria?

2. **In what contexts are decision aids for ACP currently used, and what are the limitations to their use?**
   a. Who generally facilitates the ACP decision process in which the decision aid is used?
   b. How are the decisions generated by the decision aid documented?
   c. How are the decision aid and/or its documentation transferred/communicated to health care settings where the health care activities take place?
   d. What are the implications of the combination of the health state of the person completing the decision aid, the setting in which the decision aid is completed, and whether the decisions are hypothetical or concrete?
   e. What is the legal environment and requirements for ACP for which the decision aids are used?

3. **What is the current evidence on decision aids for ACP?**
   a. What decision aids have been studied for effectiveness?
   b. What are the inclusion and exclusion criteria of people in studies of the effectiveness of decision aids?
   c. What settings were examined?
   d. What outcomes were examined?
   e. Were harms or adverse effects collected in the studies; what were they?
   f. What comparators were used to examine benefits and harms?

4. **What are the important issues raised by decision aids for advance care planning and how they are used?**
   a. What are the ethical considerations regarding using decision aids for ACP?
   b. How are people guided in choosing health care proxies?
   c. What are the implications of legal versus health care settings for ACP; do the decision aids adequately address the related concerns?
   d. What are possible areas of future research?

Methods

Technical Briefs are products of the Effective Health Care Program on important but underdeveloped topics in terms of the availability of high-quality studies. Technical Briefs provide an overview of key issues and describe available evidence. Technical Briefs do not provide synthesized evidence or grade or rate the strength of the evidence of the literature. Data presented in a Technical Brief cannot be used to develop standards or guidelines, to endorse one practice over another, or to inform policy or payment decisions, but are useful in providing direction on next steps necessary to move the topic in the direction of the development of an evidence base from which to accomplish these goals.

We integrated information from Key Informants and a literature review. In general, responses to Guiding Questions 1, 2, and 4 relied on information from Key Informants as well as gray literature and published information about decision aids and the context within which they are used. Responses to Guiding Question 3 are based on peer-reviewed, published studies that examined outcomes after the use of decision aids.

Discussion With Key Informants

We identified relevant Key Informants with the goals of efficient data collection and balanced viewpoints. We included practicing clinicians and attorneys involved in ACP, experts in medical law and medical ethics, consumer advocates, and decision aid researchers and developers. We located Key Informants from frequently listed and cited authors of relevant literature, Internet searches for possible candidates of relevant viewpoints, and nominations by other Key Informants. When we could not identify an individual to represent a specific organization, we invited the organization to nominate an individual.

We conducted semi-structured interviews with Key Informants via telephone during November 2013. Interview guides for each group of Key Informants were developed in advance. The guides are presented in Appendix A.

Gray Literature Search

We conducted a gray literature search of Federal and State government Web sites, the Ottawa Hospital Research Institute's Decision Aid Library Inventory, professional organizations, and leads from Key Informants for current decision aids available to the public and in use. Appendix C provides a list of organization Web sites searched. Resources from Web sites that provide downloadable forms for advance directive or POLST completion were excluded if they did not provide additional education or help clarify values. We also excluded resources that provided education only, without prompting action on the part of the user (e.g., ALS Association: Respiratory Decisions Guide, PBS: End of Life Dilemmas Video, Choosing Wisely: Feeding Tubes for People with Alzheimer's Disease Fact Sheet, American Health Lawyer Association: Loving Conversations Videos, Sutter VNA & Hospice: Advance Directive Intervention List).

We also searched the Internet with Google to find information on decision aids for ACP as well as on issues and controversies regarding their use. We surveyed enrolling and ongoing clinical trials though the ClinicalTrials.gov, HSRProj, and NIH RePORTER databases, and the PCORI Web site. We also searched LexisNexis for current discussions of legal/ethical considerations and controversies.

Published Literature Search

We searched MEDLINE® via OVID, the Cochrane Library, PsychINFO, and CINAHL databases through May, 2014. Exact search strategies were developed in consultation with the EPC librarian. We developed an a priori search strategy based on relevant medical subject headings (MeSH) terms and text words. The search string is provided in Appendix B. We also searched the databases using as key words the decision aids located in the gray literature.

We screened the resulting literature for relevant published articles of empirical research. For Guiding Question 3, we searched for eligible studies that examined the use of decision aids for advance care planning. We included intervention studies published in English of any sample size and any design (randomized controlled trial, controlled clinical trial, uncontrolled observational trial, and case reports and series). We excluded studies that focus on implementation science questions, including studies where the effect of a facilitator could not be separated from the effects of the decision aid. Further inclusion/exclusion criteria are provided in Table 2.

Table 2. Inclusion/exclusion criteria by PICOTS

Element	Included	Excluded
Population	Any adult potential patient, whether general or identified by disease	Pediatric patients, non-U.S. populations. Decisions must be for future care, not current care, and under consideration by the individual, not the proxy.
Interventions	Decision aids for future health states that include a behavioral prompt	• Religious or other edicts that specify what decision a patient should make (e.g., "artificial nutrition must be accepted" or "blood transfusions may not be accepted"). • An attorney's standard paragraph about preferences inserted into a health care directive that does not provide information about risks, benefits, or alternatives. • A simple form that names a health care proxy (without providing a list of powers to choose from that would be afforded to the proxy). • Health care providers' verbal recommendations. • Educational materials and research publications intended for health care professionals to help them give verbal recommendations to patients. • Educational materials that only promote the process of advance care planning, without providing information to help individuals make the decisions that are part of ACP. • Statutes, government policies, and health care institutional policy and procedure that describe and promote ACP or specify decision aids that must be used. • Advance planning for psychiatric care; decisions about treatment for a disease, not end of life decisions. Studies where the effects of the ACP facilitator could not be separated from the effects of the decision aid.
Comparators	No aid, "traditional care," education-only material	
Outcomes	Decision agreement, confidence, patient satisfaction, knowledge, comfort, uptake. May be either patient or family/caregiver	Implementation or process measures
Timing	Decisions made for future health states	Decision of current, not future or hypothetical, end-of-life decisions for current health states
Settings	Decision aids used for health care or legal settings, whether in the presence of an attorney or do-it-yourself Web sites	

Data Organization and Presentation

We abstracted data from the published literature using standardized data abstraction tables. One reviewer collected the data and assessed the evidence against the inclusion and exclusion criteria. We did not abstract actual results from the studies.

Data from the published literature were integrated with information from the gray literature and discussions with Key Informants. Responses to Guiding Questions 1 and 2 were formed with information from published narrative reviews, information in the gray literature, and Key Informant discussions. Responses to Guiding Question 3 were based primarily on peer-reviewed, published literature and may be combined with information gleaned from the gray literature (e.g., information from ongoing studies). Responses to Guiding Question 4 were informed by Key Informant discussions along with information used to address Guiding Questions 1–3.

The data are presented in narrative form (Guiding Questions 1, 2, and 4) and in evidence tables. We summarized the evidence into summary tables/plots by decision aid and its use. The tables are organized to provide descriptive details of identified decision aids and their conformance to decision aids criteria. For the criteria, we used the IPDAS instrument.[9]

Findings

Description of Existing Decision Aids for ACP

Existing Decision Aid Tools (Guiding Question 1)

The ideal ACP process is thought to occur through discussions between patients and their health care providers as part of a shared care planning process. In shared clinical decisionmaking, patients and clinicians use evidence-based knowledge, weigh options against treatment goals, and consensually arrive at a clinically prudent decision concordant with patient preferences.[21,22] Pragmatically, decision aids aim to increase patient participation and/or empowerment in decisionmaking. Although ACP is within the bounds of clinical decisionmaking, it differs from many well-studied decision processes for medical procedures (e.g., surgical or nonsurgical options for cancer) because people can complete decisionmaking with no health care provider involvement, using do-it-yourself decision aids readily available to the public. These decision aids tend to target people with only general risks of life-threatening conditions, for whom ACP may involve considering a wide range of possible future scenarios, eliciting preferred goals of care, or choosing a proxy decisionmaker.

General decision aids for ACP are often used in conjunction with tools to document the decisions, whether treatment-based, end-of-life based, or values-based. Preferences for health care can be documented in an advance directive, also known as a living will, and stored at Web sites such as MyDirectives.com. One or more proxy health care decisionmakers and their powers can be documented in a durable power of attorney for health care or as part of a more comprehensive advance directive. Health care providers can record ACP results (whether from oral discussions or in an advance directive) into health care records, a specific order (e.g., Do Not Resuscitate), or into a template most commonly called a Physician Order for Life Sustaining Treatment (POLST, found at www.polst.org). This option has the advantage of serving as standing orders.

ACP, particularly among healthy adults, occurs largely outside of clinical settings, where it is often facilitated by estate or family law attorneys or social workers rather than medical providers. Because non-medical facilitators may have limited ability to discuss health care scenarios or the success rates and consequences of life sustaining interventions, high quality decision aids would be valuable in these situations.

ACP decision aids can also address questions regarding where patients wish to die, such as in their own homes, at hospice facilities, or in skilled nursing or hospital settings. Choice of setting can have implications for available interventions. Some interventions are available only in a hospital setting (e.g., surgery), while some must be initiated in the hospital but can be managed long term at home or in a nursing facility (e.g., ventilator care). Intravenous therapies can be initiated and maintained in various settings.

Decision aids for ACP for patients with specific disease conditions can walk the undefined line between *advance* care planning and care planning. For people with predictable progressive disease (such as amyotrophic lateral sclerosis), chronic critical illness, or frailty, a structured approach to decisions in ACP often requires information regarding a person's prognosis. A patient may need to review data on life-expectancy and likelihood of pain or loss of function in order to decide for or against future life-prolonging therapies. In addition, well-informed ACP often requires intervention-specific information such as typical response and added lengths of survival. This poses significant challenges for those creating decision aids for ACP, as prognoses are often uncertain for individual patients and information on benefits of end-of-life treatments are rarely available for specific populations that match a patient's circumstances.

Tables 3a and 3b describe generally available tools for ACP. These tools were identified through the gray literature search and by Key Informants. The list is not exhaustive. It captures the more commonly known decision aids, or those relatively easy to find online via common search engines. These tools vary in the degree to which they meet the three criteria of our working ACP decision aids definition, based on the IPDAS instrument criteria:[8,9] an education component, a structured approach to thinking about the choices a patient faces, and a way for those choices to be communicated. Tools in both tables are indexed by decision and degree to which the tool meets the three decision aid criteria.

Table 3a describes 10 general ACP decision tools for healthy older adults with an undetermined illness trajectory. The most popular ACP topics covered by tools in Table 3a include: designating a health agent or proxy decisionmaker (7/10), value clarification and desire for comfort care at the end of life (7/10), information on living wills or advance directives (5/10), conversation prompts for talking to loved ones or physicians about wishes (5/10), and general preferences for various life sustaining treatments (4/10). Other topics considered included: organ and tissue donation (2/10), identification of states worse than death (1/10), and preference for treatment location (1/10). Many of the general tools targeted at healthy older adults address multiple ACP topics (mode, four topics per tool). The breadth of the general tools is great, but the depth is compromised. This is evidenced in the degree to which the tools meet decision aid criteria. Most tools provide low or medium levels of education and decisional structure. They provide communication of decisions because they are often attached to an advanced directive or living will, or prompt completing one.

In contrast, Table 3b includes eight tools for individuals with a life limiting illness for which the decision trajectory is often more clearly defined. These tools are distinct from the general population tools in Table 3a because they are more likely to focus on one ACP topic (6/8) and to be designed by a shared decisionmaking organization (6/8). These tools are more likely to meet decision aid criteria because the information they provide is more precise and targeted at specific decisions. However, two tools in Table 3b (Looking Ahead: Choices for Medical Care When You're Seriously Ill and the PEACE SERIES) are similar to the tools in Table 3a; they cover a number of general topics without a lot of depth. Although the tools in Table 3b are more likely to be designed by decisionmaking organizations (such as the Informed Medical Decisions Foundation and Healthwise) and to be reviewed by the Ottawa Hospital Research Institute, the tools do not appear in the published, peer reviewed literature. A disconnect exists between the gray literature tools and decision aids and the empirical literature.

Table 3a. Examples of general ACP tools publicly available on the World Wide Web

Organization/ Name of Tool	Topics Addressed by Tool								Developer's Description	DA Criteria			URL
	Living Will or AD	Health Agent	Life Sustaining Treatments-Multiple	States Worse than Death	Organ and Tissue Donation	Conversation Prompts	Treatment Location	Comfort Care Value Identification		Provides Education	Structured Approach	Decision Communication	
ADVault Inc./ MyDirectives	X	X	X		X	X	X	X	MyDirectives is the first completely online advance directive that is secure, legal, easy to understand, and free. MyDirectives is also the first advance care platform to receive "meaningful use" certification from HHS so that hospitals may be eligible for incentive payments from Medicare and Medicaid under the American Recovery and Reinvestment Act when using this technology	M	M	H	www.mydirectives.com/?MyD
Aging with Dignity / The Five Wishes	X	X	X					X	The Five Wishes document helps individuals express care options and preferences. The advance directive meets the legal requirements in most states and is available in 20 languages for a nominal fee.	L	L	M	www.agingwithdignity.org/five-wishes.php
American Bar Association / Consumer's Toolkit for Health Care Advance Planning		X	X	X	X	X		X	The tool kit does not create a formal advance directive for you. Instead, it helps you do the much harder job of discovering, clarifying, and communicating what is important to you in the face of serious illness.	L	M	M	www.americanbar.org/groups/law_aging/resources/consumer_s_toolkit_for_health_care_advance_planning.html
Caring Connections: National Hospice and Palliative Care Organization / End-of-Life Decisions	X	X	X						This booklet addresses issues that matter to us all, because we will all face the end of life. Advance directives are valuable tools to help us communicate our wishes about our future medical care.	M	L	L	www.caringinfo.org/files/public/brochures/End-of-Life_Decisions.pdf

Table 3a. Examples of general ACP tools publicly available on the World Wide Web (continued)

Organization/ Name of Tool	Topics Addressed by Tool								Developer's Description	DA Criteria			URL
	Living Will or AD	Health Agent	Life Sustaining Treatments-Multiple	States Worse than Death	Organ and Tissue Donation	Conversation Prompts	Treatment Location	Comfort Care Value Identification		Provides Education	Structured Approach	Decision Communication	
Center for Practical Bioethics/Caring Conversations	X	X	X					X	Caring Conversations equips you with the tools you will need to communicate your wishes when you can no longer speak for yourself and advocate on your own behalf. The workbook includes a Durable Power of Attorney for Healthcare Decisions form and a Healthcare Treatment Directive form.	L	M	M	www.cpbmembers.org/documents/Caring-Conversations.pdf
Coalition for Compassionate Care of California/ Advance Care Planning Conversation Guide						X			The ACP conversation guide provides suggestions on how to raise the issue, responses to concerns your loved one might express, and questions to ask.	L	L	L	http://coalitionccc.org/wp-content/uploads/2014/01/Advance-Care-Planning-Conversation-Guide1.pdf
Conversation Project, Institute for Healthcare Improvement/ Conversation Starter Kit and How to Talk to Your Doctor						X		X	The Conversation Project is dedicated to helping people talk about their wishes for end-of-life care with family members and physicians.	M	M	M	http://theconversationproject.org/wp-content/uploads/2013/01/TCP-StarterKit.pdf
Engage with Grace/ Engage with Grace: The One Slide Project						X			The One Slide Project was designed with one simple goal: to help get the conversation about end of life experience started. The idea is simple: Create a tool to help get people talking. One Slide, with just five questions on it. Five questions designed to help get us talking with each other, with our loved ones, about our preferences.	L	L	L	www.engagewithgrace.org/

Table 3a. Examples of general ACP tools publicly available on the World Wide Web (continued)

Organization/ Name of Tool	Topics Addressed by Tool								Developer's Description	DA Criteria			URL
	Living Will or AD	Health Agent	Life Sustaining Treatments-Multiple	States Worse than Death	Organ and Tissue Donation	Conversation Prompts	Treatment Location	Comfort Care Value Identification		Provides Education	Structured Approach	Decision Communication	
Georgia Health Decisions/CRITICAL Conditions Planning Guide	X	X			X			X	The CRITICAL Conditions Planning Guide walks you through advance care planning, beginning with meaningful conversations among your family members and resulting in the legal documentation of your preferences.	L	M	M	www.critical-conditions.org/preview.html
Lancashire and South Cumbria Cancer Services Network/Preferred Priorities for Care (PPC)		X					X	X	The PPC document is recommended to help identify patient preferences for end-of-life care and prevent unwanted hospital admissions at the end of life.	L	L	M	www.dyingmatters.org/sites/default/files/user/images/PPC%20final%20document.pdf
The Regents of the University of California/ PREPARE	X	X				X		X	PREPARE is an interactive Web site serving as a resource for families navigating medical decisionmaking. PREPARE is a program that can help you: make medical decisions for yourself and others, talk with your doctors, get the medical care that is right for you.	M	H	H	https://www.prepareforourcare.org/

L=low, M=medium, H=high

Table 3b. Examples of ACP tools for those with serious or advanced illness publicly available on the World Wide Web

Organization/ Name of Tool	Topics Addressed by Tools									Developer's Description	DA Criteria			URL
	Living Will or AD	Health Agent	Life Sustaining Treatment	Life Support & CPR	Kidney Dialysis	Pain	Artificial Nutrition & Hydration	Conversation Prompts	Treatment Location	Comfort Care Value Identification		Provides Education	Structured Approach	Decision Communication	
American College of Physicians/ PEACE Series		X				X		X		X	The Consensus Panel project convened a second group of experts to develop patient education materials and Web content on end-of-life care for patients with serious or advanced illness. ACP's End-of-Life Care PEACE Series patient education brochures are available in print or to view online.	M	L	L	www.acponline.org/patients_families/end_of_life_issues/peace/
Healthwise/ Should I have artificial hydration and nutrition							X			X	This decision aid is for patients considering artificial hydration and nutrition if or when they are no longer able to take food or fluids by mouth.	H	H	M	https://print.healthwise.net/kaiser/kpisg/PrintTableOfContents.aspx?token=kpisg&localization=en-us&version=&docid=tu4431
National Cancer Institute at the NIH/Questions to Ask Your Doctor About Advanced Cancer								X			If you learn that you have advanced cancer, you may have choices to make about care and next steps. When you meet with your doctor, consider asking some of the following questions.	L	L	L	www.cancer.gov/cancertopics/cancerlibrary/questions/advanced-cancer
Healthwise/ Should I stop kidney dialysis?					X					X	This decision aid helps patients with kidney failure who have been undergoing dialysis, and for whom kidney transplantation is not possible, decide whether to continue kidney dialysis, which will allow you to live longer or stop kidney dialysis, which will allow death to occur naturally.	H	H	M	https://print.healthwise.net/kaiser/kpisg/PrintTableOfContents.aspx?token=kpisg&localization=en-us&version=&docid=tu6095

Table 3b. Examples of ACP tools for those with serious or advanced illness publicly available on the World Wide Web (continued)

Organization/ Name of Tool	Topics Addressed by Tools										Developer's Description	DA Criteria			URL
	Living Will or AD	Health Agent	Life Sustaining Treatment	Life Support & CPR	Kidney Dialysis	Pain	Artificial Nutrition & Hydration	Conversation Prompts	Treatment Location	Comfort Care Value Identification		Provides Education	Structured Approach	Decision Communication	
Healthwise/ Should I receive CPR and life support				X						X	This decision aid helps patients with serious or advanced illness decide whether or not to receive CPR and be put on a ventilator if heart or breathing stops.	H	H	M	https://print.healthwise.net/kaiser/kpisg/Print/PrintTableOfContents.aspx?token=kpisg&localization=en-us&version=&docid=tu2951
Healthwise/ Should I stop treatment that prolongs my life?			X							X	This decision aid helps patients with serious or advanced illness decide whether to stop treatment that prolongs life and instead receive only hospice care, or to continue treatment that prolongs life.	H	H	M	https://print.healthwise.net/kaiser/kpisg/Print/PrintTableOfContents.aspx?token=kpisg&localization=en-us&version=&docid=tu1430
Informed Medical Decisions Foundation/ Looking Ahead: Choices for Medical Care When You're Seriously Ill	X	X	X							X	This program is for people with a serious illness that is or may become life threatening. This program is also for family members and caregivers. The program describes different types of medical care, such as palliative care and hospice care, and reviews various types of advance directives.	M	L	M	During report preparation this decision aid became proprietary under a different organization. See www.healthdialog.com/Utility/News/PressRelease/14-01-17/Health_Dialog_and_the_Informed_Medical_Decisions_Foundation_Restructure_Longstanding_Relationship.aspx#

Table 3b. Examples of ACP tools for those with serious or advanced illness publicly available on the World Wide Web (continued)

Organization/ Name of Tool	Topics Addressed by Tools										Developer's Description	DA Criteria			URL
	Living Will or AD	Health Agent	Life Sustaining Treatment	Life Support & CPR	Kidney Dialysis	Pain	Artificial Nutrition & Hydration	Conversation Prompts	Treatment Location	Comfort Care/ Value Identification		Provides Education	Structured Approach	Decision Communication	
Ottawa Patient Decision Aid Research Group/When you need extra care, should you receive at home or in a facility?									X		This decision aid helps patients with serious or advanced illness decide whether they would like to receive care at home or in a facility	H	H	H	http://decisionaid.ohri.ca/docs/das/Place_of_Care.pdf

L=low, M=medium, H=high

Context in Which ACP Decision Aids Are Used (Guiding Question 2)

Decision aids can better standardize the ACP process across facilitators or improve its efficiency. A variety of health care professionals, legal advisors, clergy, and even trained volunteers are available to facilitate ACP. When no decision aid is used, the facilitator's personal knowledge and biases have more opportunity to influence decisions. The facilitator's employer may also have financial incentives that influence which decision aids are used. For example, when a facilitator is employed or sponsored by a health care insurer, the business model of the insurer would possibly lead to decision aids that are biased towards limitations of treatment. Attorneys may find decision aids in ACP helpful given their lack of health care training. On the other hand, when a decision aid is used, the biases of its creators become relevant.

While attorneys typically charge an hourly rate for facilitation of ACP, reimbursement for health care provider time related to ACP is much more complex. Physicians, nurse practitioners, and physician assistants can select billing codes based on the amount of time they spend counselling patients for ACP, but only when such counselling takes up the majority of face-to-face time of an encounter. In all other cases, these providers as well as nurses, social workers, and chaplains who assist with ACP must consider facilitation of ACP as part of the overhead expense of the health care practice or institution, without separate or specific reimbursement. Several attempts to add ACP facilitation as a separate type of service into Medicare reimbursement policies have failed in Congress. This limitation in reimbursement inhibits many efforts to expand ACP, and reduces the willingness of health care institutions to invest in decision aid development or purchase, except where such tools improve efficiency of ACP or advance institutions' desired outcomes of ACP (e.g., fewer deaths in hospital).

Promotion and facilitation of ACP has been strongest in health crisis settings, when the "advance" part of ACP is hours to days. For example, the iconic SUPPORT study focused on decisionmaking in the intensive care unit.[17,23,24] Similarly, ACP is heavily promoted in regulations for nursing homes, with advocacy for decisionmaking to take place at or near admission. Alternatively, shared decisionmaking for ACP can happen earlier in the course of an illness but after the patient develops a relationship with a trusted health care professional. Decision aids can be useful in all of these contexts, but most patients can best use such a tool before crises and with a strong patient-clinician relationship.

The POLST, which translates preferences resulting from ACP into a medical order, is intended primarily for those who have life expectancies less than 1 to 2 years. The form may be placed in a health care record or given to a patient to have available at home. A POLST provides explicit instructions from the signing physician to other physicians (e.g., in an emergency room), nurses, emergency medical personnel, and others. The POLST provides some legal and regulatory authorization to clinicians to provide or withhold emergency treatments without need for further discussion or need to obtain and review an advance directive. About one-third of States have statutes related to POLST. Decision aids to assist with the creation of a POLST form may be specific to the types of interventions addressed in a POLST, such as cardiopulmonary resuscitation, intubation for respiratory failure, and feeding tubes.

Hospitals, nursing homes, and some other health care programs are mandated to ask patients whether they have a health care directive. Recent clarifications in regulations require that nursing homes seek to determine patient preferences and enact processes to honor those preferences. Yet, no Federal or State mandates address the content or structure of ACP discussions; every State has statutes related to the documentation of preferences in health care directives.

Because State law governs almost all issues related to end-of-life care, decision aids for ACP should be consistent with a State's laws and regulations. For example, some States require that in order for a proxy to have authority regarding withholding or withdrawing a feeding tube, that preference must be explicitly stated in a health care directive, while other States grant a proxy discretion on that issue. Thus, an excellent decision aid for use in one State may mislead a patient's effort to document preferences in another State. This limits the ability of organizations to develop decision aids for ACP that contain enough detail for effective completion of an ACP process. Web sites such as FindLaw (http://statelaws.findlaw.com/minnesota-law/minnesota-durable-power-of-attorney-laws.html) and Caring Connections (http://www.caringinfo.org/i4a/pages/index.cfm?pageid=3289) provide examples of available resources.

Evidence Map

Current Evidence of ACP Decision Aids (Guiding Question 3)

As noted, the tools and decision aids found through gray literature search and consultation with Key Informants (Tables 3a and 3b) were not uncovered in the published literature search. The literature search yielded 363 articles. (Figure 2) Only 15 studies met the criteria for the correct patient population, intervention, and outcome measures.[25-38] Studies that were excluded due to patient population included those that examined the use of end-of-life decision aids with families of chronic and critically ill newborns, children, and adolescents. The majority of studies were excluded based on lack of a decision aid intervention. These studies described or evaluated how patient, surrogate, or physician characteristics (race, health literacy, disability), structural components (culture of intensive care unit, education of physicians), economic incentives, or ethical considerations affect the end-of-life communications and care decisions, but did not include the use of a decision aid. Also excluded were studies that focused on decision theory or studies in which the primary outcomes of interest were the psychometric properties of a decision tool or aid. One study was excluded because the decision tool was for a research advance directive.[39] A protocol for a randomized control trial was also excluded, as outcome information is not yet available.[40] An additional study was located by

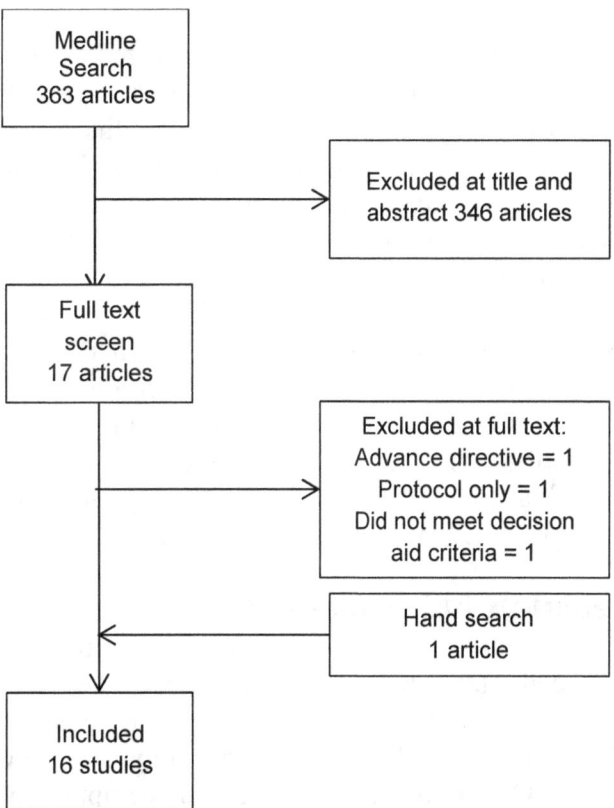

Figure 2. Article flow diagram

searching for decision aids identified in the gray literature search, bringing the total included studies to 16.

We identified an additional 10 ongoing studies from ClinicalTrials.gov and HRS-Proj databases (see Appendix C). However, 6 of the 10 trials appear to assess videos produced by ACP Decisions.

Evaluating the effectiveness of ACP decision aids is a relatively recent phenomenon, closely linked to the creation of criteria for patient decisionmaking in general. Fourteen of the 16 included studies were published within the last 5 years.

Details of the included studies are summarized in Tables 4 and 5 and discussed in the next sections.

Study Designs

Of the 16 studies, 9 were RCTs[25,27,29,34,35,37,38,41,42] and 7 were case-series.[26,28,30-33,36] Two RCTs used a multiple treatment design.[25,27] We could not determine whether harms information was systematically collected in many studies. Three studies included patient levels of stress and anxiety or hope to assess whether the use of the aid had increased distress as a side effect of using the tool.[28,33,34]

Patient Populations

The patient populations included in studies of decision aids for advance care planning include both patients with serious or advance illness and community-dwelling older adults or older adults without serious or advanced illness. This distinction is important: the valuation of health states changes with increasing age and experience of illness.[10] Physicians treating a patient with advanced cancer may want to use a tool that has been studied in or designed for that population. Of the 16 included studies: 9 studies evaluated decision aids on community-dwelling older adults or older adult populations,[25-27,29,31,32,35,37,38] 6 evaluated decision aids on patients with serious or advanced illness,[30,33,34,36,41,42] and 1 evaluated its decision aid on both general and disease specific populations.[28] The nongeneral populations studied included patients with advanced cancers,[28,33,36,42] patients undergoing cardiac surgery,[34] and patients with amyotrophic lateral sclerosis (ALS),[30] and inpatient palliative care.[41] Many studies had additional inclusion criteria for age,[25-27,34,35,37,38] language comprehension,[25,29,32,35,38] level of cognitive functioning,[25-27,30,35-38] availability of proxy,[27,34,37] and presence of target condition.[30,33,34,36] One study required participants to have access to a computer.[42]

Decision Aid Modalities

Decision aids took several forms: self-directed computer program or Web page,[28-31,42] enhanced information,[25] scenario-based AD,[27] value-based AD,[27] video depiction of patients with advanced disease,[26,35,36,38] disease prognosis statistics,[33] structured interview,[34] interactive CD-ROM,[32] and a DVD with an accompanying booklet.[41] Eleven unique decision aids were studied. One of these, the self-directed computer program entitled "Making Your Wishes Known," is directed at individuals rather than organizations, and is publicly available at https://www.makingyourwishesknown.com/default.aspx. Similarly, "Looking Ahead: Choices for Medical Care When You're Seriously Ill" is publicly available in streaming video format on the Informed Medical Decisions Foundation Web site: http://www.informedmedicaldecisions.org/imdf_decision_aid/choosing-medical-care-for-the-seriously-ill/.[a] However, the video-based aids produced by the nonprofit foundation, ACP Decisions, (http://www.acpdecisions.org/videos/), and the structured Patient Centered Advance Care Planning interview are not for general public use; these tools are marketed toward specific health systems' beneficiaries. The former is a commercial product, primarily designed for health care organizations; the latter was created by such an organization. The cancer prognosis statistics decision aid is available in the original article appendix,[33] and similar tools are available to physicians on the Adjuvant Web site (http://www.adjuvantonline.com/index.jsp). Three tools were described in the original articles but are not easily found in the public domain: the interactive CD-ROM,[32] the enhanced information aid,[25] a Web site intervention in pilot stage,[42] the scenario-based AD, and the value-based AD.[27]

Comparators

The seven case-series studies had no comparison group by design.[26,28,30-33,36] The comparison groups for the RCTs and controlled trials included control groups that received usual care,[41] groups that received usual care in the same format as the intervention arm,[42] groups that did not complete an advance directive,[27] groups that were given advance directive forms without education or with written educational materials,[29,34] or verbal and vignette description of conditions (without video enhancement).[25,35,37,38] Green et al. (2011) provides an example of a clear description of usual care for advance directives: "This standard packet provides basic education about advance directives, sections for assigning a surrogate decisionmaker and outlining specific end-of-life wishes, along with instructions on how to complete the form. But it does not include values clarification exercises, education about medical conditions/treatments, or a decision support tool for assisting in decisionmaking" (page 84).[29] This description is consistent with the definition of a decision aid used in this technical brief to identify appropriate gray literature tools.

Decision Aid Outcomes

Table 5 summarizes the assessed outcomes examined from the reviewed tools. Primary study outcomes include: patient satisfaction with decision aid or perceived helpfulness of decision aid (13/16), clarity regarding patient preference for comfort care (7/16), patient knowledge of advance directives or disease process (11/16), decisional conflict or confidence in decision (5/16), effect of tool on patient stress (3/16), patient/proxy decision concordance (2/16), effect of tool on patient hope (2/16), patient/physician decision concordance (1/16), preference stability over time (1/16), and advance directive documentation and scheduled consultation with palliative care (1/16). The studies report that while tools were generally well received and interpreted as helpful by patients, the effect of a decision aid on a patient's care choices and the communication of these choices to a health proxy or attending physician is mixed.

The nature of the outcomes that can be tested for ACPs depends on where the patient is on the continuum in Figure 1. Measures like "extending the patient's autonomy" can be tested only when the decision is imminent. Only three included studies evaluated the ability of the decision aid to improve surrogate decisionmaking or to increase the likelihood a patient's wishes being honored at the end of life.[27,31,34]

---

[a] During report preparation this decision aid became proprietary under a different organization. See http://www.healthdialog.com/Utility/News/PressRelease/14-01-17/Health_Dialog_and_the_Informed_Medical_Decisions_Foundation_Restructure_Longstanding_Relationship.aspx#

Some studies examined outcomes that can be assessed contemporaneously with the intervention, such as: whether participants felt their surrogates better understood their wishes, that the tools provided comfort to their surrogates,[27] whether the use of a decision aid was helpful to patients,[26,28-30,32,33,35-38] reduced decisional conflict,[25,41,43] or increased patient knowledge of end-of-life decisions.[26,32-34,36-38,41]

In the following paragraphs we describe how satisfaction, decisional conflict, and education were assessed in the included studies, and we highlight validated tools with potential for standardizing evaluation.

Satisfaction/Helpfulness

Among the included studies, the most commonly evaluated outcome was satisfaction or perceived helpfulness of tool.[26,28-30,32,33,35-38] A related outcome is the likelihood of a patient recommending the tool to a friend or person with the same health condition.[35-38] Five studies evaluating the same tools, the ACP Decision videos, all reported percentages of participants in the intervention group finding the tool "very helpful" or "somewhat helpful" and the percentage of participants in the intervention group who would "definitely" or "probably" recommend the tool.[26,35-38] One questionnaire simply asked if the information was helpful (yes or no).[33] Matlock et al. (2011)[41] was the only study to mention modifying an established shared decisionmaking acceptability tool. In addition to helpfulness of the decision aid and patient willingness to recommend it to a friend, the shared decisionmaking acceptability tool asks about the information provided including the amount, clarity, and viewpoint or neutrality[41]

Decisional Conflict/Sense of Control

Three included studies used different versions of the Decisional Conflict scale.[25,41,43] The validated Decisional Conflict scale assesses patients' perceptions of uncertainty, modifiable factors contributing to the uncertainty, and ultimate satisfaction with choice.[43] Hossler et al. (2011) adapted a self-determination scale developed by Pellino et al. (1998)[44] to evaluate a distinct but related outcome: the patient's sense of control.[30] Items on this scale included: "I can plan for my future medical needs," "I can effectively communicate my wishes to my doctors," and "I have the power to affect what happens to me in the future."[30]

Knowledge

The educational assessments varied by target population. A video intervention focused on care choices for CPR and ventilation among terminal cancer patients asked six true/false questions including: "Most cancer patients who survive CPR and are placed on a breathing machine have very few complications from these procedures," and "Most cancer patients that get CPR in the hospital survive and get to leave the hospital."[36] Murphy et al. (2000) also tested knowledge using the true or false format; the items included: "Draw up AD once you are ill to ensure accuracy," "AD are only used to refuse treatment," and "Avoid second guessing of your AD treatment preference."[32] Another study targeting cancer patients asked yes/ no questions (e.g., "Can this person with cancer in the bones and lymph nodes be cured by medical treatment?"), and asked participants to predict the likelihood of their cancer shrinking by half.[33] Three studies measured participant perceptions of improved knowledge. Two studies used a Likert type scale to assess whether the participant believed knowledge was improved after using tool.[37,38] One study provided percentages of participants mentioning educational outcomes after using the decision aid.[26]

Care Intensity Consistent With Patient Preferences

Five included studies evaluated the effect of the decision aid on increasing the likelihood a participant would choose less care.[25,26,35-38] According to the IPDAS Collaboration, no clear treatment choice should apply to everyone; the best choice for end-of-life care is the amount of treatment that is consistent with a patient's values.[9]

Table 4. ACP decision aid studies

Study	Study Design	Population	Tool Name	Modality	Comparator
Volandes et al., 2012[36]	Case series	80 patients with advanced cancers	ACP Advanced Cancer Video	Video	Patients served as own control, before and after viewing video (all subjects received verbal description of care choices)
Deep et al., 2010[26]	Case series	120 community dwelling older adults	ACP Advanced Dementia Video	Video	Patients served as own control, before and after viewing video (all subjects received verbal description of care choices)
Volandes et al., 2009[37]	Randomized controlled trial	14 community dwelling older adults and their surrogates	ACP Advanced Dementia Video	Video	Patients randomized to verbal description only or verbal description with video decision aid
Volandes et al., 2009 (BMJ)[38]	Randomized controlled trial	200 community dwelling older adults	ACP Advanced Dementia Video	Video	Patients randomized to verbal description only or verbal description with video decision aid
Volandes et al., 2011[35]	Randomized controlled trial	76 community dwelling older adults	ACP Advanced Dementia Video	Video	Patients randomized to verbal description only or verbal description with video decision aid
Smith et al., 2011[33]	Case series	27 patients with advanced cancers	Adjuvant	Disease prognosis and probability statistics	Patients served as own control, before and after using decision aid
Allen et al., 2008[25]	Randomized controlled trial	78 community dwelling older adults		Enhanced information on life-sustaining treatment risks, benefits, and alternatives	Patients randomized to medical information stimuli and the Life Support Preferences / Predictions Questionnaire (LSPQ) vignettes, or LSPQ vignettes only
Ditto et al., 2001[27]	Randomized controlled trial	401 community dwelling older adults	Health Care Directive (HCD) Valued Life Activities Directive (VLA)	Scenario-based advanced directive Value-based advanced directive	Patients randomized HCD no discussion, HCD with discussion, VLA no discussion, VLA with discussion, or no advance directive
Matlock et al., 2011[41]	Randomized controlled trial	51 inpatient palliative care patient or their decisionmaker	Looking Ahead: Choices for medical care when you're seriously ill	Booklet and DVD	Patients randomized to usual palliative consult services or usual care and the decision aid
Murphy et al., 2000[32]	Case series	31 community dwelling older adults	Making Decisions About Health Care	Interactive CD-ROM	Patients served as own control, before and after using decision aid
Green et al., 2009[28]	Case series	50 community dwelling older adults 34 patients with cancer	Making Your Wishes Known: Planning Your Medical Future	Self-directed computer program	Patients reported satisfaction and enhanced knowledge with use of aid.

Table 4. ACP decision aid studies (continued)

Study	Study Design	Population	Tool Name	Modality	Comparator
Green et al., 2011[29]	Randomized controlled trial	121 community dwelling older adults 121 medical students	Making Your Wishes Known: Planning Your Medical Future	Self-directed computer program	Medical students and patients dyads were randomized to usual care or decision aid arms.
Hossler et al., 2011[30]	Case series	17 patients with amyotrophic lateral sclerosis (ALS)	Making Your Wishes Known: Planning Your Medical Future	Self-directed computer program	Patients served as own control, before and after using decision aid
Levi et al., 2011[31]	Case series	19 community dwelling older adults	Making Your Wishes Known: Planning Your Medical Future	Self-directed computer program	Evaluation of decision aid's ability to appropriately guide physician making
Song et al., 2005[34]	Randomized controlled trial	32 patients undergoing cardiac surgery and their surrogate	Patient-Centered Advance Care Planning	Structured interview	Patients randomized to usual advanced directive care (information packet and access to pastoral care facilitator) or decision aid
Vogel et al., 2013[42]	Randomized controlled trial	53 women with ovarian cancer were enrolled, 35 completed the study		Self-directed computer program	Patients randomized to a control Web site with usual care information or the decision aid

Table 5. Outcomes examined by ACP decision aid studies

Study	Population	Modality	Tool Name	Satisfaction / Perceived Benefits of Tool	Care Intensity Consistent with Patient Preferences	AD or Disease Knowledge	Preference Stability Over Time	Reduce Decisional Conflict	Patient / Proxy Concordance	Patient / Doctor Concordance	Patient Hope	Patient Stress or Anxiety	AD Documentation / Palliative Consult
Volandes et al., 2012[36]	Patients with advanced cancers	Video	ACP Advanced Cancer Video	+	NE	+							
Deep, et al., 2010[26]	Community dwelling older adults	Video	ACP Advanced Dementia Video	+	+	+							
Volandes et al., 2009[37]	Community dwelling older adults	Video	ACP Advanced Dementia Video	+	+	+							
Volandes et al., 2009 (BMJ)[38]	Community dwelling older adults	Video	ACP Advanced Dementia Video	+	+	+	+						
Volandes et al., 2011[35]	Community dwelling older adults	Video	ACP Advanced Dementia Video	+	+								
Smith et al., 2011[33]	Patients with advanced cancers	Disease prognosis and probability statistics	Adjuvant	+		+					NE	NE	
Allen et al., 2008[25]	Community dwelling older adults	Enhanced Information on life-sustaining treatment risks, benefits, and alternatives			+AA* White			+					
Ditto et al., 2001[27]	Community dwelling older adults	Scenario-based AD Value-based AD	Health Care Directive (HCD) Valued Life Activities Directive (VLA)	+	NE				NE				
Matlock et al., 2011[41]	Inpatient Palliative Care	Booklet and DVD	Looking Ahead: Choices for medical care when you're seriously ill	+		NE		NE					
Murphy et al., 2000[32]	Community dwelling older adults	Interactive CD-ROM	Making Decisions About Health Care	+		+							

Table 5. Outcomes examined by ACP decision aid studies (continued)

Study	Population	Modality	Tool Name	Satisfaction / Perceived Benefits of Tool	Care Intensity Consistent with Patient Preferences	AD or Disease Knowledge	Preference Stability Over Time	Reduce Decisional Conflict	Patient / Proxy Concordance	Patient / Doctor Concordance	Patient Hope	Patient Stress or Anxiety	AD Documentation / Palliative Consult
Green et al., 2009[28]	Community dwelling older adults, Patients with cancer	Self-directed computer program	Making Your Wishes Known: Planning Your Medical Future	+		+					NE	NE	
Green et al., 2011[29]	Community dwelling older adults, Medical students	Self-directed computer program	Making Your Wishes Known: Planning Your Medical Future	+		+							
Hossler et al., 2011[30]	Patients with amyotrophic lateral sclerosis (ALS)	Self-directed computer program	Making Your Wishes Known: Planning Your Medical Future	+		+							
Levi et al., 2011[31]	Community dwelling older adults	Self-directed computer program	Making Your Wishes Known: Planning Your Medical Future					+		+			
Song et al., 2005[34]	Patients undergoing cardiac surgery	Structured interview	Patient-Centered Advanced Care Planning	NE		NE		+	+			NE	
Vogel et al., 2013[42]	Patients with advanced ovarian cancer	Self-directed computer program		NE				NE					NE

AD= advance directive. NE=no effect found. AA=African American. +The study reported positive findings for that outcome. − The study reported negative findings for that outcome. Blank cell=not evaluated.
*African Americans differed from whites in preferences for receiving comfort care versus life sustaining care.

Evaluating ACP Decision Aids

The IPDAS Collaboration has developed criteria for evaluating the quality of a decision aid (http://ipdas.ohri.ca/IPDAS_checklist.pdf). In Table 6, we use the broad categories from the IPDAS checklist to identify the index question and briefly evaluate the quality of the decision aid content and development for the decision aid tools. We evaluate the identified decision aids from Table 3 and the published decision aids presented in Table 4.

An important component for the IPDAS decision aid evaluation is having an index decision. In evaluating ACP decision aids, we excluded tools with the main goal of prompting discussion of individual values for end-of-life care with loved ones and physicians. These questions, while important, do not equate to index decisions. Only three tools from the published literature could be evaluated using the IPDAS standards (Adjuvant, Making Your Wishes Known: Planning Your Medical Future, and Looking Ahead: Choices For Medical Care When You're Seriously Ill). The ACP Decisions videos depicted a woman with advanced Alzheimer's disease, but did not focus on a decision. A few of the decision aids were not publicly available.[25,27,32] The Respecting Choices, Patient-Centered Advanced Care Planning interview is proprietary and used only by those completing proprietary training modules.

Compared with condition-specific aids, general decision aid tools that helped people choose a proxy and make advanced directive decisions provided less information about the index decisions. For the most part, advanced planning tools targeted at the general public were less likely to help people deliberate on their decision using a structured process. Two notable exceptions are the interactive online resources, PREPARE and MyDirectives. Both tools help patients deliberate and communicate their decisions, while providing considerable information and video examples for each decision.

The decision aid tools that focus on only one decision point are more likely to provide high levels of information and help the user deliberate or decide. Five of the decision-specific tools have been previously reviewed by the Ottawa Patient Decision Aid Research (OPDAR) using the IPDAS criteria. The content criteria can be evaluated by an individual viewing the tool, but the development criteria are less apparent on most of the organization Web sites. The five tools reviewed by OPDAR had this information available in their decision aid summaries, available on their Web site: http://decisionaid.ohri.ca/index.html.

Applying the IPDAS criteria to the decision aid tools highlights the general lack of effectiveness information. An effective decision aid leads to decisions (whether made by the patient or surrogate) that are informed and consistent with the decisionmaker's values. Few tools on the OPDAR Web site meet all effectiveness criteria. Generally available decision aids do not provide information to evaluate whether effectiveness has been assessed. For the decision aids found in the published effectiveness literature, the outcome measures are not effectiveness measures, as measured by the IPDAS, but measures of satisfaction and desire for comfort care over life-sustaining treatment. If comfort care is the choice that is consistent with the informed consumer's values and wishes, then the tool is effective. However, some informed consumers will have value systems that lead them to choose life sustaining care.

Key informants specified a set of important criteria for assessing decision aids. The first criterion is whether the decision aids are balanced, informing but not selling particular philosophical stances or specific decisions. The second criterion is whether decision aids present narratives of people who have gone through the experiences, particularly if several voices provide different perspectives to enhance the decision aid balance. The third criterion is making core facts available to reduce the likelihood of overestimating the value of interventions and the odds of good outcomes. Finally, decision aids should present relevant facts effectively and accessibly.

Table 6. Evaluating ACP decision aids

Name of Tool	Index Decision				Decision Aid Content							Decision Aid Development				Effectiveness
	Selection of Health Proxy	Preference for Multiple ACP Decisions	Preference for a Specific Life-Prolonging Treatment	Preference for Place of Care	Provide Information	Present Probabilities	Clarify Patient Values	Guide Decision Deliberation	Guide Decision Communication	Present Balanced Information	Systematic Development	Cite Scientific Evidence	Disclose COI	Use Plain Language	Decisions are Informed and Value Based
The Five Wishes	X	X			L		X		X					X	
Consumer's Toolkit for Health Care Advanced Planning	X	X			M		X		X						
Caring Connections: End of Life Decisions	X	X			M		X								
Caring Conversations	X	X			M		X	X	X					X	
CRITICAL Conditions Planning Guide	X	X			M		X	X	X					X	
"Thinking Ahead" – GSF Advance Care Planning Discussion	X	X		X			X		X					X	
PREPARE	X	X			H		X	X	X	X	X				
Should I have artificial hydration and nutrition?			X		H	X	X	X	X	X	X	X	X	X	M
Should I stop kidney dialysis?			X		H	X	X	X	X	X	X	X	X	X	M
Should I receive CPR and life support?			X		H	X	X	X	X	X	X	X	X	X	M
Should I stop treatment that prolongs my life?			X		M	X	X	X	X	X	X	X	X	X	M
Looking Ahead: Choices for Medical Care When You're Seriously Ill	X	X			M		X				X				
When you need extra care, should you receive it at home or in a facility?			X		M		X	X	X	X	X		X	X	
Adjuvant			X		H	X	X	X	X	X	X		X	X	M
Looking Ahead: Choices for Medical Care When You're Seriously Ill	X	X			M	X	X		X		X		X	X	
Making Your Wishes Known: Planning Your Medical Future	X	X			M		X	X	X	X	X		X		M

X=item was identified as present or met. L= Low; M = Medium; H = High.

Summary and Implications

Important Issues Raised by the Technology (Guiding Question 4)

Key Informants raised several important issues regarding decision aids and their place in ACP.

As laid out in the findings, decision aids serve two broad functions in ACP: (1) to identify a proxy decisionmaker, and (2) to decide in advance on preferences for care in specific situations. Many Key Informants and some ACP Web sites promote a staged approach to ACP with the goals and outcomes varying by the individual's particular circumstances. Only those with advanced illness or at high risk of catastrophic health events are encouraged to seek specific information on their condition and options for life-sustaining treatments, and then encouraged to name a health care proxy decisionmaker and make sure that person is aware of care preferences. All others with less certain future health needs are simply encouraged to choose and document a health care proxy decisionmaker. Several Key Informants noted the difficulty of determining the information that will best serve people's needs unless the target audience is clearly defined, which is often easiest for disease-specific tools. A staged approach to ACP, based on how hypothetical the decision aid index question is and the level of uncertainty about the care choices to consider, would help guide the important education components, appropriate evaluation, and convergence with care planning.

Several Key Informants suggested that for people with serious or chronic critical illnesses, ACP functions best when integrated into overall care plans. Then, advanced care decisions can be discussed in the context of other care options and based on the options available in the chosen care setting, since services vary by location (e.g., nursing home versus hospital). Care decisions can imply a willingness to move to a more (or less) intensive environment (e.g., do not hospitalize instructions). Without explicit information about which services are available in various settings, patients may express preferences for or against therapies and for or against settings that turn out to be incompatible. Or they may express preference to decline certain therapies on a mistaken assumption that such an intervention can only be offered in the hospital.

For those with established conditions, ACP decisions need to be based, in part, on knowledge of prognosis. High-quality decision aids could inform patients about their prognosis and allow them to consider potential implications for health care decisions. Ideally, patients would be given information on the expected natural history of their condition(s) as well as the efficacy of various life-sustaining interventions to change the course or experience of illness, and potential harms. Clinical and administrative databases (i.e., Big Data) could provide current and continually updated information or prognosis and treatment efficacy in advanced illness. A challenge remains, however, when it comes to creating interactive or patient-specific tools that can help patients and clinicians estimate probabilities of intervention benefits in various circumstances near the end of life. Prognosis and planning is even more challenging for diseases with less certain trajectories (for example, heart disease or dementia versus metastatic cancer). This makes it hard for providers to know what to talk about when, and for designers of decision support materials to know what to include in a decision aid.

The need for such information in decision aids becomes clear in situations where patients and families anticipate future difficulties with maintenance of oral nutrition. The likelihood of such a problem varies across diseases, such as Alzheimer's, Parkinson's, strokes, ALS, and esophageal disorders. The benefits of medical nutrition, such as enteral feeding through a gastrostomy tube, also vary significantly depending on the cause of poor oral intake. Without data-rich decision aids, patients with early Alzheimer's might mistakenly believe there is therapeutic benefit from enteral feeding (none is found in multiple studies). Meanwhile, those with primary swallowing disorders might mistakenly extrapolate information from populations with dementia and underestimate the benefits of oral nutrition for their condition.

The way questions are posed by decision aids can affect responses. Several Key Informants noted discomfort with some ACP video images of people with advanced illness. They noted that the images could be alarming to people of generally good health who are far from experiencing such diminished health states, and thus bias viewers towards less care than they may otherwise have chosen. Providing accurate information and frames that portray a realistic range of health state experiences is challenging, and a "good balance" may very well be in the eye of the beholder. Other Key Informants found video vignettes particularly important for engaging people in the decisionmaking process for ACP, helping them envision possible future health states they may have otherwise avoided. However, the use of heuristics for decisionmaking tends to increase as decisional complexity increases, such as when a person's emotional intensity state is high.[44]

Key Informants suggested taking the "A" out of ACP by making ACP an ongoing process rather than a one-time decision to be documented. Certainly, decisions need to be revisited as a patient's condition deteriorates. The Gold Standards Framework Tool "Thinking Ahead – GSF Advance Care Planning Discussion" guide is one example of a tool intended as a dynamic document to be adapted and reviewed as needed. However, other Key Informants stressed that the urgent need to have people complete at least one ACP should take precedence over creating decision aids to support dynamic ACPs.

Several Key Informants noted that decision aids need to be tolerant of the many philosophical perspectives that people may bring to the process. In a country as diverse as the United States, decision aids should be culturally and spiritually sensitive to traditions and supportive of nuanced decisions. Decision aids should be flexible to the process rather than focused solely on the outcome.

Key Informants expressed concern over the use of computer-based decision aids and ACP documentation tools due to potential access problems should there be exclusive or over-reliance of Web-based tools. This concern also applied to decision aids and tools not free and easily available to the public. Certain patient populations without easy access to computer resources are disadvantaged. One way to provide ACP decision aids to vulnerable populations would be through ACP bringing the decision aid materials or resources to the patients.

Key Informants differed on the role of specialized facilitators and who would best fulfill such a role. Differences could concern the specific professional training (e.g., social workers and nurses versus clergy versus physicians versus lawyers) or might reflect specialized training in ACP facilitation regardless of discipline. The latter approach highlights the skills the facilitator brings to the encounter rather than the role. Yet, the greater the demand for special status, the greater the tendency for problems with access issues due to increased costs. As a prime skill regardless of who fills the role, Key Informants noted the ability to respect the decision made, whether or not the facilitator agrees with it.

Although providers are often the automatic default facilitators, several Key Informants noted that physicians are often the most challenged to facilitate conversations a difficulty they attributed to various causes, from personal difficulty with talking about dying and end-of-life decisions when their training and motivation is toward curing and prolonging life to more traditional concerns regarding patriarchal attitudes. To this, we add the practical barriers that hinder physicians from engaging in ACP conversations, such as time constraints, financial disincentives, and the absence of effective strategies for promoting ACP conversations.

Although most ACP tools include choice of proxy decisionmaker, Key Informants noted a lack of decision aids designed to help people choose a proxy well. However, a couple of attempts have been made. For example, Caring Connections provides some links on their Web page, but does not directly take up the task. Key Informants further noted that in-depth conversations between people and their proxies are needed to establish clarity about personal values and outcome preferences. These conversations give the proxy a sense of confidence for representing the patient when end-of-life decisions must finally be made. One Key Informant noted that voice recordings of the patient's preferences and values can be a powerful way to make the patient's wishes "real" during the difficult times.

Ultimately, decision aids provide a structure that allows people to deeply consider and document their preferences and support important relationships. A well-considered and communicated preference helps doctors feel assured and comfortable about the ethics of providing or withholding treatments that affect survival. Effective decision aids help provide closure to family and loved ones who will live with the consequences.

Next Steps

Future directions for efforts to improve ACP decision aids fall into three categories.

1. Research is needed:
   - Well-designed, validated tools that are easily accessible, readable, understandable, and appropriate to patients across various settings working with various facilitators. Some progress has been made, but much remains to be done. A broad array of tools may be needed to meet the needs of the broad array of professionals, in different settings, and at various stages of the Figure 1 map.
   - Comparing various decision aids, including patient and provider satisfaction, impact on preferences stated, and efficiency of the ACP processes. These studies might include attention to who facilitates decisions and how.
   - Better ways of presenting risk information to patients, more individualized predictive models for life expectancy that can be incorporated into ACP decision aids, and understanding if the risk information improved patient decisionmaking. Alternatively, tools could also be developed to better help patients cope with or adapt to uncertainty as an inherent part of ACP and life course.
   - Effectiveness of various end-of-life interventions in different clinical populations. This information would improve the educational components of ACP decision aids.
   - Ways to design decision aids that enable patients to work backwards from their preferred site of care to then decide which therapies they might accept in that setting (because location of care is sometimes a dominant preference in ACP).
   - Ways to evaluate decision aids for the context within which they are intended to be used, because professionals supporting ACP may include clinicians, lawyers, social workers, and clergy (or none).

All of the research next steps would be furthered by agreement on a core set of outcomes to assess the effectiveness of the decision aids. Table 7 provides a possible core set derived from the IPDAS criteria and outcomes used in the empirical literature. The listed outcomes diverge from the IPDAS set with outcomes related to the surrogate decisionmaker's role in ACP. Serious consideration should also be given to what "harms" should be consistently collected in ACP decision aid research as well.

Table 7. Potential outcome measure by stage

Outcome	Stage of Health / Illness			
	Healthy	Potentially Life Threatening Illness	Life Threatening Illness or Event	Hospice or Frail Elderly
Extending autonomy			X	X
Wishes honored		?	X	X
Improved decisionmaking	X	X	X	X
Improved communication	X	X	X	X
Patient/provider concordance	X	X	X	X
Patient/surrogate concordance	X	X	X	X
Surrogate understanding of patient's wishes	X	X	X	X
Surrogate comfort	X	X	X	X
Satisfaction	X	X	X	X
Helpfulness	X	X	X	X
Decisional conflict	X	X	X	X
Sense of control	X	X	X	X
Improved emotional state/hope/reduction of anxiety		X	X	X
Knowledge	X	X	X	X
Care intensity consistent with preferences	X	X	X	X

2. Training of current or future facilitators of ACP (health professionals, attorneys, clergy, social workers) is needed regarding:
   - Shared decisionmaking, using decision aids.
   - Use of decision aids, to reduce variation in the process of ACP.
   - Value of decision aids, to improve clarity of verbal and written communication.
   - More understanding of how the background of the decision facilitator affects the decision processes.

3. Use of social media and other technologies provide further opportunities to improve decision aid development.
   - Create decision aids that provide personal narratives based on patient experiences in various health conditions and after receiving life prolonging therapies. Several of the decision aid resources presented here have started this process. More could be accomplished using social media to democratize the process of sharing and collecting patient experiences.
   - Social media and other big data sources may also allow access to more fine-grained individualized information to help improve not only prognostic abilities, but also to illuminate what choices people have made and the resulting course. People like to know how other people have chosen and behaved.

References

1. Kaldjian LC, Curtis AE, Shinkunas LA, et al. Goals of care toward the end of life: a structured literature review. American Journal of Hospice & Palliative Medicine. 2008 Dec-2009 Jan;25(6):501-11. PMID: 19106284.
2. Heyland DK, Dodek P, Rocker G, et al. What matters most in end-of-life care: perceptions of seriously ill patients and their family members. . Canadian Medical Association Journal. 2006;174(5):627-33. PMID: 16505458.
3. Emmanuel L, Scandrett KG. Decisions at the end of life: have we come of age? BMC Medicine. 2010;8:57. PMID: 20932275.
4. Daaleman TP, VandeCreek L. Placing religion and spirituality in end-of-life care. JAMA. 2000;284(19):2514-7. PMID: 11074785.
5. Balboni TA, Balboni M, Enzinger AC, et al. Provision of spiritual support to patients with advanced cancer by religious communities and associations with medical care at the end of life. JAMA Internal Medicine. 2013;173(12):1109-17. PMID: 23649656.
6. Wilkinson A, Wenger N, Shugarman LR. Literature review on advance directives. 2007.
7. Witherspoon GS. What I learned from Schiavo. Hastings Center Report. 2007;37:17-20. PMID: 18179100.
8. O'Connor AM, Stacey D, Entwistle V, et al. Decision aids for people facing health treatment or screening decisions (Cochrane Review). Chichester, UK. 2004.
9. Elwyn G, O'Connor AM, Bennett C, et al. Assessing the quality of decision support technologies using the international patient decision aid standards instrument (IPDASi). PLoS One. 2009;4(3):e4705. .
10. Dolan P. Addressing misconception in valuing health. Expert Review of Pharmacoeconomics & Outcomes Research. 2013;13(1):2-4. PMID: 23402439.
11. Ubel PA, Loewenstein G, Schwarz N, et al. Misimagining the unimaginable: the disability paradox and health care decision making. Health Psychology. 2005;24(4 Suppl):S57-62. PMID: 16045420.
12. Sackett DL, Torrance GW. The utility of different health states as perceived by the general public. Journal of Chronic Diseases. 1978;31(11):697-704. PMID: 730825.
13. Kind P, Dolan P. The effect of past and present illness experience of the valuations of health states. Medical Care. 1995;33(4 Suppl):AS255-63. PMID: 7723454.
14. Stacey D, Legare F, Col N, et al. Decision aids for people facing health treatment or screening decisions. 2014.
15. Advance Care Planning, Preferences for Care at the End of Life: Research in Action. Rockville, MD. March 2003. www.ahrq.gov/research/findings/factsheets/aging/endliferia/index.html.
16. Virmani J, Schneiderman LJ, Kaplan RM. Relationship of advance directives to physician-patient communication. Archives of Internal Medicine. 1994;Apr 25;154(8):909-13. PMID: 8154954.
17. Teno J, Lynn J, Wenger N, et al. Advance directives for seriously ill hospitalized patients: effectiveness with the patient self-determination act and the SUPPORT intervention. Journal of the American Geriatrics Society. 1997;45(4):500-7. PMID: 9100721.
18. Teno J, Licks S, Lynn J, et al. Do advance directives provide instructions that direct care? Journal of the American Geriatrics Society. 1997;45:508-12. PMID: 9100722.
19. Bradley EH, Rizzo JA. Public information and private search: evaluating the Patient Self-Determination Act. Journal of Health Politics, Policy, and Law. 1999;24(2):239-73. PMID: 10321357.
20. Coppola KH, Ditto PH, Danks JH, et al. Accuracy of primary care and hospital-based physicians' predictions of elderly outpatients' treatment preferences with and without advance directives. Archives of Internal Medicine. 2001;161(431-40). PMID: 11176769.
21. Montori VM, Gafni A, Charles C. A shared treatment decision-making approach between patients with chronic conditions and their clinicians: The case of diabetes. Health Expectations. 2006;9(25-36). PMID: 16436159.
22. Charles C, Gafni A, Whelan T. Shared decision-making in the medical encounter: What does it mean? (Or it takes at least two to tango). Social Science and Medicine. 1997;44(681-692). PMID: 9032835.
23. Halliday S, Witteck L. Decision-making at the end-of-life and the incompetent patient: a comparative approach. Medicine & Law 2003;22(3):533-42. PMID: 14626885.
24. Covinsky KE, Goldman L, Cook EF, et al. The impact of serious illness on patients' families. SUPPORT Investigators. Study to Understand Prognoses and Preferences for Outcomes and Risks of Treatment. JAMA. 1994;Dec 21;272(23):1839-44. PMID: 7990218.

25. Allen RS, Allen JY, Hilgeman MM, et al. End-of-life decision-making, decisional conflict, and enhanced information: race effects. Journal of the American Geriatrics Society. 2008;Oct;56(10):1904-9. PMID: 18775035.
26. Deep KS, Hunter A, Murphy K, et al. "It helps me see with my heart": how video informs patients' rationale for decisions about future care in advanced dementia. Patient Education & Counseling. 2010;Nov;81(2):229-34. PMID: 20194000.
27. Ditto PH, Danks JH, Smucker WD, et al. Advance directives as acts of communication: a randomized controlled trial. Archives of Internal Medicine. 2001;Feb 12;161(3):421-30. PMID: 11176768.
28. Green MJ, Levi BH. Development of an interactive computer program for advance care planning. Health Expectations. 2009;Mar;12(1):60-9. PMID: 18823445.
29. Green MJ, Levi BH. Teaching advance care planning to medical students with a computer-based decision aid. Journal of Cancer Education. 2011;Mar;26(1):82-91. PMID: 20632222.
30. Hossler C, Levi BH, Simmons Z, et al. Advance care planning for patients with ALS: feasibility of an interactive computer program. Amyotrophic Lateral Sclerosis. 2011;May;12(3):172-7. PMID: 20812887.
31. Levi BH, Heverley SR, Green MJ. Accuracy of a decision aid for advance care planning: simulated end-of-life decision making. Journal of Clinical Ethics. 2011;22(3):223-38. PMID: 22167985.
32. Murphy CP, Sweeney MA, Chiriboga D. An educational intervention for advance directives. Journal of Professional Nursing. 2000;Jan-Feb;16(1):21-30. PMID: 10659516.
33. Smith TJ, Dow LA, Virago EA, et al. A pilot trial of decision aids to give truthful prognostic and treatment information to chemotherapy patients with advanced cancer. The Journal of Supportive Oncology. 2011;Mar-Apr;9(2):79-86. PMID: 21542415.
34. Song MK, Kirchhoff KT, Douglas J, et al. A randomized, controlled trial to improve advance care planning among patients undergoing cardiac surgery. Medical Care. 2005;Oct;43(10):1049-53. PMID: 16166875.
35. Volandes AE, Ferguson LA, Davis AD, et al. Assessing end-of-life preferences for advanced dementia in rural patients using an educational video: a randomized controlled trial. Journal of Palliative Medicine. 2011;Feb;14(2):169-77. PMID: 21254815.
36. Volandes AE, Levin TT, Slovin S, et al. Augmenting advance care planning in poor prognosis cancer with a video decision aid: a preintervention-postintervention study. Cancer. 2012;Sep 1;118(17):4331-8. PMID: 22252775.
37. Volandes AE, Mitchell SL, Gillick MR, et al. Using video images to improve the accuracy of surrogate decision-making: a randomized controlled trial. Journal of the American Medical Directors Association. 2009;Oct;10(8):575-80. PMID: 19808156.
38. Volandes AE, Paasche-Orlow MK, Barry MJ, et al. Video decision support tool for advance care planning in dementia: randomised controlled trial. BMJ. 2009;338:b2159. PMID: 19477893.
39. Stocking CB, Hougham GW, Danner DD, et al. Empirical assessment of a research advance directive for persons with dementia and their proxies. Journal of the American Geriatrics Society. 2007;Oct;55(10):1609-12. PMID: 17714461.
40. Bravo G, Arcand M, Blanchette D, et al. Promoting advance planning for health care and research among older adults: a randomized controlled trial. BMC Medical Ethics. 2012;13:1. PMID: 22221980.
41. Matlock D, Keech T, McKenzie M, et al. Feasibility and acceptability of a decision aid designed for people facing advanced or terminal illness: a pilot randomized trial. Health Expectations. 2011. PMID: 22032553.
42. Vogel RI, Petzel SV, Cragg J, et al. Development and pilot of an advance care planning website for women with ovarian cancer: a randomized controlled trial. Gynecol Oncol. 2013;Nov;131(2):430-6. PMID: 23988413.
43. Song MK, Sereika SM. An evaluation of the Decisional Conflict Scale for measuring the quality of end-of-life decision making. Patient Education & Counseling. 2006;Jun;61(3):397-404. PMID: 15970420.
44. Arana J, Leon C, Hanemann M. Emotions and decision rules in discrete choice experiments for valuing health care programmes for the elderly. Journal of Health Economics. 2008;May;27(3):753-69. PMID: 18241944.

Appendix A. Interview Guides for Key Informants

Questions for experts/researchers/provider organizations/practicing clinicians
   a. What decision aids do you use in advance care planning?
   b. What specific ACP tools and aids characterize your program? (May we see them?)
   c. What do you see as the strengths and weaknesses of the decision aids you have used? The barriers and facilitators of using the decision aids?
   d. Gray literature: which professional organizations are important to consult regarding:
      i. Tools
      ii. Preliminary study findings
   e. Review/comment on definitions of ACP and decision aid models.
   f. What types of research are needed most? What outcomes? What designs? When should outcomes be measured (length of followup)?
   g. What format works best in your experience?
   h. Which health care directive form do you prefer?

Questions for patient advocates, families, caregivers
   a. What information do patients need to know when planning advance care?
   b. Does that information change based on your level of health?
   c. What do you view as the advantages/disadvantages of advance planning?
   d. How did the decision aid help with the planning process?

Questions for ethicists/clergy/law
   a. What do you consider important ethical considerations that need to be addressed with regard to ACP and decision aids?
   b. How do decision aids help or change the dynamics of the ACP process itself, and, if conducted as a dialogue, discussions between patients, family members, and providers?
   c. What information do you believe is most needed by people considering ACP?
   d. What kinds of research would be most useful? What outcomes?
   e. To what extent should the health care professional facilitating the conversation give advice (person as decision aid)?

Appendix B. Published Literature Search Strategy

We searched MEDLINE using the algorithm listed below. We adjusted the algorithm to also search the Cochrane Library, PsychINFO, and CINAHL databases.

Database: Ovid MEDLINE® <1946 to August Week 4 2013> Search Strategy:

1	exp Advance Care Planning/
2	exp Advance Directives/
3	"advanced care plan*".ti.
4	"advance* care plan*".m_titl.
5	(advance* adj2 directive*).ti.
6	"living will*".m_titl.
7	"end of life".mp.
8	exp Decision Support Techniques/
9	exp Decision Support Systems, Clinical/
10	decision aid*.mp.
11	decision tool*.mp.
12	decision support.mp.
13	instrument*.ti,ab.
14	intervention*.ti,ab.
15	program*.ti,ab.
16	exp *Decision Making/
17	13 or 14 or 15
18	15 and 16
19	8 or 9 or 10 or 11 or 12 or 18
20	1 or 2 or 3 or 4 or 5 or 6 or 7
21.	19 and 20

Appendix C. Organization Web sites Searched for Gray Literature

Organization
Aging with Dignity
Allina Health
ALS Association
American Bar Association
American College of Physicians
Caring Connections
Center for Advanced Illness Coordinated Care, National Hospice and Palliative Care Organization
Center for Practical Bioethics
Coalition for Compassionate Care of California
Conversation Project, Institute for Healthcare Improvement
Deathwise
Engage with Grace
Georgia Health Decisions
Gold Standards Framework
Gundersen Health System, Respecting Choices
Healthwise
Henry Ford Health System
Honoring Choices Minnesota
Informed Medical Decisions Foundation
Lancashire and South Cumbria Cancer Services Network
Lifecare Directives, LLC
National Cancer Institute at the NIH
National Hospice and Palliative Care Organization
National POLST Paradigm Task Force
Ottawa Patient Decision Aid Research Group
PBS Religion & Ethics Newsweekly
Renal Palliative Care Initiative
Robert Wood Johnson Foundation, Promoting Excellence in End of Life Care
Sutter VNA and Hospice
The Huntington's Disease Workgroup of Promoting Excellence in End-of-Life Care
The Regents of the University of California

Appendix D. Evidence Tables

Table D1. Gathered examples of commonly used or accessible decision aids

Name of Tool/ Organization	Target Population	Description	Purpose of Tool	Tool Format
The Five Wishes/ Aging with Dignity	General planning before a medical event or terminal illness	The Five Wishes document helps individuals express care options and preferences. The advance directive meets the legal requirements in most states and is available in 20 languages for a nominal fee.	AD education and completion	Order hard copy or complete online. Educational DVDs available.
Consumer's Toolkit for Health Care Advanced Planning/ American Bar Association	General planning before a medical event or terminal illness	The toolkit does not create a formal advance directive for you. Instead, it helps you do the much harder job of discovering, clarifying, and communicating what is important to you in the face of serious illness.	AD education Clarify values	Downloadable guide
End-of-Life Decisions/ Caring Connections	General planning before a medical event or terminal illness	This booklet addresses issues that matter to us all, because we will all face the end of life. Advance directives are valuable tools to help us communicate our wishes about our future medical care.	AD education	Downloadable guide
Caring Conversations/ Center for Practical Bioethics	General planning before a medical event or terminal illness	Caring Conversations equips you with the tools you will need to communicate your wishes when you can no longer speak for yourself and advocate on your own behalf. The workbook includes a Durable Power of Attorney for Healthcare Decisions form and a Healthcare Treatment Directive form.	AD education and completion Conversation guide	Downloadable guide
Advanced Care Planning - Conversation Guide/ Coalition for Compassionate Care of California	General planning before a medical event or terminal illness	The ACP conversation guide provides suggestions on how to raise the issue, responses to concerns your loved one might express, and questions to ask.	Conversation guide or prompts	Downloadable guide

Table D1. Gathered examples of commonly used or accessible decision aids

Name of Tool/ Organization	Target Population	Description	Purpose of Tool	Tool Format
Conversation Starter Kit and How to Talk to Your Doctor/ Conversation Project, Institute for Healthcare Improvement	General planning before a medical event or terminal illness	The Conversation Project is dedicated to helping people talk about their wishes for end-of-life care with family members and physicians.	Conversation guide or prompts	Online resource and downloadable guides
Engage with Grace: The One Slide Project/Engage with Grace	General planning before a medical event or terminal illness	The One Slide Project was designed with one simple goal: to help get the conversation about end-of-life experience started. The idea is simple: create a tool to help get people talking. One Slide, with just five questions, is designed to help get us talking with each other and with our loved ones about our preferences.	Conversation guide or prompts	Web page with downloadable slide
CRITICAL Conditions Planning Guide/ Georgia Health Decisions	General planning before a medical event or terminal illness	The CRITICAL Conditions Planning Guide walks you through advance care planning, beginning with meaningful conversations among your family members and resulting in the legal documentation of your preferences.	AD education and completion Conversation guide	Order hard copy or download
Preferred Priorities for Care (PPC)/ Lancashire and South Cumbria Cancer Services Network	General planning before a medical event or terminal illness	The PPC document is recommended to help identify patient preferences for end-of-life care and prevent unwanted hospital admissions at the end of life.	Document patient wishes	Downloadable guide
PREPARE/The Regents of the University of California	General planning before a medical event or terminal illness	PREPARE is an interactive Web site serving as a resource for families navigating medical decisionmaking. PREPARE is a program that can help you: make medical decisions for yourself and others, talk with your doctors, and get the medical care that is right for you.	AD education and completion Conversation guide	Video/interactive online resource
PEACE Series/ American College of Physicians	Patient with serious/ advanced illness	The Consensus Panel project convened a second group of experts to develop patient education materials and Web content on end-of-life care. ACP's End-of-Life Care PEACE Series patient education brochures are available in print or to view online.	Conversation guide or prompts	Downloadable brochures
Should I have artificial hydration and nutrition?/Healthwise	Patients considering artificial hydration and nutrition if or when they are no longer able to take food or fluids by mouth	This decision aid helps patients decide whether or not to have artificial hydration and nutrition.	Education, value determination, document decision	Online resource

Table D1. Gathered examples of commonly used or accessible decision aids

Name of Tool/ Organization	Target Population	Description	Purpose of Tool	Tool Format
Questions to Ask Your Doctor About Advanced Cancer/ National Cancer Institute at the NIH	Patients with advanced cancer	If you learn that you have advanced cancer, you may have choices to make about care and next steps. When you meet with your doctor, consider asking some of these questions.	Conversation guide or prompts	Online resource
Should I stop kidney dialysis?/Healthwise	Patients with kidney failure who have been undergoing dialysis, and for whom kidney transplantation is not possible	This decision aid helps patients decide whether to continue kidney dialysis, which will allow you to live longer, or stop kidney dialysis, which will allow death to occur naturally.	Education, value determination, document decision	Online resource
Should I receive CPR and life support?/ Healthwise	Patients with serious/ advanced illness	This decision aid helps patients decide whether or not to receive CPR and be put on a ventilator if heart or breathing stops.	Education, value determination, document decision	Online resource
Should I stop treatment that prolongs my life?/ Healthwise	Patients with serious/ advanced illness	This decision aid helps patients decide whether to stop treatment that prolongs life and instead receive only hospice care or not to stop treatment that prolongs life.	Education, value determination, document decision	Online resource
Looking Ahead: Choices for Medical Care When You're Seriously Ill/Informed Medical Decisions Foundation	Patients with serious/ advanced illness	This program is for people with a serious illness that is, or may become, life threatening. This program is also for family members and caregivers. The program describes different types of medical care, such as palliative care and hospice care, and reviews various types of advance directives.	Education, value determination	Available as a DVD, a booklet, and a Web-based program
When you need extra care, should you receive it at home or in a facility?/Ottawa Patient Decision Aid Research Group	Patients with serious/ advanced illness	This decision aid helps patients decide whether they would like to receive care at home or in a facility	Education, value determination, document decision	Downloadable pdf

Table D2. List of identified relevant studies from trial registries

Trial # (Registry)	Trial Name	Investigators / Study Sponsor / Collaborators
NCT01190488 (ClinicalTrials.gov- Completed)	Feasibility of an advanced care decision aid among patients and physicians	D Matlock / University of Colorado, Denver
NCT01325519 (ClinicalTrials.gov- Recruiting)	A prospective randomized trial using video images in advanced care planning in seriously ill hospitalized patients	AE Volandes / Massachusetts General Hospital
NCT01527331 (ClinicalTrials.gov- Recruiting)	A prospective trial using video images in advance care planning in hospitalized seriously ill patients with advanced cancer	AE Volandes / Massachusetts General Hospital / Stanford University
NCT01589120 (ClinicalTrials.gov- Recruiting)	Using videos to facilitate advance care planning for patients with heart failure (VIDEO-HF)	AE Volandes / Massachusetts General Hospital / University of Colorado, Denver, Vanderbilt University, South Shore Hospital, Brigham and Women's Hospital, Boston Medical Center
NCT01445145 (ClinicalTrials.gov- Completed)	An exploratory study of the use of Five Wishes as a tool for advanced care planning in young adults with metastatic, recurrent, or progressive cancer or HIV infection	L Wiener / National Cancer Institute
NCT01105806 (ClinicalTrials.gov- Ongoing, not recruiting)	Cardiopulmonary resuscitation (CPR) video to enhance advance care planning in advanced upper gastrointestinal cancer patients	E O'Reilly / Memorial Sloan-Kettering Cancer Center / Massachusetts General Hospital, Mount Sinai Hospital, New York
NCT01391429 (ClinicalTrials.gov- Unknown)	Testing a video decision support tool to supplement goals-of-care discussions	M Paasche-Orlow, A Volandes / Boston Medical Center
NCT01653938 (ClinicalTrials.gov- Recruiting)	A trial of a CPR video in heart failure patients	A Volandes / Massachusetts General Hospital
HSRP20122281 (HRS-Proj – Ongoing)	Using videos to facilitate advance care planning for patients with heart failure	A Volandes / Massachusetts General Hospital / John D. Stoeckle Center for Primary Care Innovation, National Heart, Lung, and Blood Institute
HSRP20104051 (HSRProj – Ongoing)	Improving end-of-life care for cancer patients with video decision aids	A Volandes / Massachusetts General Hospital / Agency for Healthcare Research and Quality

Appendix E. Examples of Advanced Care Planning Tools That Did Not Meet Definition of Decision Aid

Organization	Name of Tool	Target Population	Description	Purpose of Tool	Tool Format	Accessed	URL
Gold Standards Framework	'Thinking Ahead' – GSF Advance Care Planning Discussion	General planning before a medical event or terminal illness	Advance Statement should be used as a guide, to record what the patient DOES WISH to happen, to inform planning of care. This is a 'dynamic' planning document to be adapted and reviewed as needed and is in addition to Advanced Directives, Do Not Resuscitate plan, or other legal document.	Document patient wishes and prompt discussion	Downloadable form	Gold Standards Framework	http://www.goldstandardsframework.org.uk/advance-care-planning
ALS Association	ALS Respiratory Decisions	Patients with ALS	This pamphlet is designed to help the person with ALS make the choice or choices appropriate for them and their family. This information is for your education only and is not intended to replace the medical advice of your personal physician or other members of your health care team.	Document patient wishes and prompt discussion	Downloadable guide	The ALS Association Jim "Catfish" Hunter Chapter	http://webnc.alsa.org/site/DocServer/brochure_RespiratoryDecisions.pdf?docID